Feeling Good
a beginner's guide

by

Anthea Wheal

Green Magic

Feeling Good: a beginner's guide © 2014 Anthea Wheal
All rights reserved
No part of this book may be used or reproduced in any form without permission of the author, except in the case of quotations in articles and reviews

Green Magic
5 Stathe Cottages
Stathe
Somerset TA7 0JL
England

info@greenmagicpublishing.com
www.greenmagicpublishing.com

ISBN 978 0 9566197 7 8

Green Magic

Contents

Introduction 5
Essentials 7
Art 11
Becoming Pagan 13
Being Enthusiastic 15
Being Green 17
Bird Watching 19
Breathing 21
Clothes and Fashion 23
Collecting 25
Computing Skills 27
Cooking and Eating In 29
Dowsing with a Pendulum 31
Dreaming 33
Driving 35
Eating out 37
Exercise and Playing Games 39

Family	41
Food	43
Friends	45
Gardening	47
Genealogy	49
Health	51
Hobbies	53
Holidays	55
Lifestyle	57
Medication	59
Meditation	61
Music	63
Optimism	65
Pets	67
Photography	69
Poetry	71
Random Acts of Kindness	73
Reading	75
Running	77
Singing	79
Sleep	81
Spirituality	83
Star Gazing	85
Supporting a Team	87
Travel	89
Using a Tarot Pack	91
Walking	93
Watching Old Movies	95
Work and Job	97
Write a Book	99
Yoga	101
Zen	103

Introduction

Almost everyone would like to be able to say that they feel good. There are many different ways of saying this, and many expressions that we all use every day to convey the best frame of mind and state of health. It's much easier to be able to say 'I feel good' when all is going smoothly – when you have the job you always wanted, money in the bank, the members of your family are in good health and your friends are all around you.

Life is not like that all the time, unfortunately! So, when your idea of happiness and contentment is checked, or ruined, by events that unexpectedly occur (as they do!) then we all need a way to step around, through or over the event that has knocked everything out of kilter.

Sometimes it's not enough to just put on a brave face or vow to carry on regardless with a smile pinned to your lips. At these moments (or months, or years) when things have gone wrong, it's necessary to break the stasis of not feeling how you would like to and to get into a zone of interest and enjoyment. This nearly always means finding something new to do. Don't call it a hobby or pastime, as that may feel old fashioned and dated – you need something that holds your interest and gives a new insight into how things work for you.

This book contains a collection of ideas, activities and add-ons for your days that can help to make the positive change and help you become the person you want to be. There will be at least one thing here that makes it worthwhile, and finding it and doing it will make you feel good.

There is a difference between being happy and feeling good. There is a difference between having no worries and feeling good. There is a difference between feeling okay and feeling good. There is a difference between feeling well and feeling good. Feeling good is a health, ethics, diet, emotion and outlook thing. Having money may make you feel happy, but it might not make you feel good!

Feeling good is really about being properly ready, and equipped, to cope with the challenges you will meet. Feeling good means having a bunch of skills to get you through a problem or around an obstacle.

Essentials

This is a list of things you should make sure you do in your life to avoid the feeling of missing out! It's made up of the top five regrets felt by people on their deathbeds. It was compiled by Bonnie Ware, who is a palliative nurse. It's much more important to do what you feel is right, rather than what you feel other people think is right. This is a truth on many levels and should be given serious thought, and acted on by seizing chances when they come along, without hesitation. Here are the things to consider in your life, above all else, to make you feel good.

I wish I'd had the courage to live a life true to myself, not the life others expected of me.

This was the most common regret of all. When people realise that their life is almost over and look back on it clearly, it is easy to see how many dreams have gone unfulfilled. Most people had not honoured even a half of their dreams and died knowing that this was due to choices they had made, or not made. Health brings a freedom very few realise, until they no longer have it.

I wish I hadn't worked so hard.

This came from every male patient. They missed their children's youth and their partner's companionship. Women also spoke of this regret, but as most were from an older generation, many of the female patients had not been breadwinners. All of the men deeply regretted spending so much of their lives on the treadmill of a work existence.

I wish I'd had the courage to express my feelings.

Many people suppressed their feelings in order to keep peace with others. As a result, they settled for a mediocre existence and never became who they were truly capable of becoming. Many developed illnesses relating to the bitterness and resentment they carried as a result.

I wish I had stayed in touch with my friends.

Often, they would not truly realise the full benefits of old friends until their dying weeks and it was not always possible to track them down. Many had become so caught up in their own lives that they had let golden friendships slip by over the years. There were many deep regrets about not giving friendships the time, and effort, that they deserved. Everyone misses their friends when they are dying.

I wish that I had let myself be happier.

This is a surprisingly common one. Many did not realise until the end that happiness is a choice. They had stayed stuck in old patterns and habits. The so-called 'comfort' of familiarity overflowed into their emotions, as well as their physical lives. Fear of change had them pretending to others, and to themselves, that they were content, when deep within, they longed to laugh properly and have silliness in their life again.

Art

The idea of art is routed in creativity. Any work of art shows a desire to live and shows a viewer something that's been made that its maker thought worthwhile. You don't have to be a Picasso or Leonardo. Do a pencil drawing for your eyes only, or just use a biro to doodle on the corner of a piece of paper. It's not so much what you do but the fact that you are doing it that will give you a lift. You can, of course, get yourself down to an art shop or stationers and buy a few bits and pieces and set up a little corner to do some studied work. There's no need to spend a bunch of cash to get going.

There is a popular feeling that art is very specialised, but this is not true – anyone can do it. There is no limit to how your art can turn out and it doesn't matter who it is for, apart from you.

This is about creative painting rather than house painting or decorating. A couple of paintbrushes, a glass of water and some watercolour paints are a good place to start this very enjoyable and cheap creative flow. Make sure you are painting for yourself only and not trying to show off a skill. You may have to shut yourself away!

It is easy to feel that your work is no good. It may be the case that you have no natural skill at art. This does not matter. It's all about pushing paint about on the paper and enjoying the colours and mixing them together, and trying out little ideas on a corner of a piece of paper. Do not try to create an image of anything particular to start with, just see what colours you like and how the paint comes off the brush onto the page. You can always just do a pencil rough or half sketch and see what happens if you just colour it in. Once dry you can go over it again, or just throw it away and no-one will ever know.

Maybe you would rather do a bit of modelling with clay. All you need is a few basic kitchen utensils, a knife and a teaspoon. Collage is also fun to do and can be made up from any fragments of material and paper scraps – you just need glue and a piece of cardboard.

Sign up for an evening class at your local college. It is great to get out of yourself and see what other people are doing. The inspiration for any art is buried inside us all and whether you try it or not, it's a personal decision and not one necessarily based on skill!

Inspiration is not frequently studied but it is, by its nature, beyond control.

Becoming Pagan

An important part of life is not to follow leaders and religious institutions because, although offering reassurance, they are hardly guaranteed to make you feel good. The answer for many is to formulate your own view of the world and how it works, and becoming Pagan is well worth checking out. We are not talking about anything out of the ordinary, as Pagans (literally 'country lovers' in old Greek) have been around for thousands of years. To be Pagan, all you need do is get into a frame of mind that tells you that what is a natural and simple way of life cannot be all wrong.

Find out what time the sun rises and sets and check out what the moon phase is. Then see what season you are in. If it's summer then the Solstice can be celebrated simply by finding a time to mark with a fire in the garden, a special meal, a trip to the country, or a walk up your favourite hill. If it's winter then you have the shortest day to celebrate and make a bit of a feast and fun. It's about getting into the rhythm of the earth and its yearly cycle of events.

When you start looking into it, you will become aware that it is what your ancestors did for thousands of years. It puts you in the zone which, when inhabited, makes it easier to see what is going on and how things work. Once you get into the actual rhythm of the world, you are participating in the truly important events in human life. You will be moving in the same direction as the universe.

You do not have to dance naked under a full moon or join a coven. You can just follow a path that works for you and honours the earth and nature. Being Pagan is about living and responding to the pattern of life.

If you are a rebel and wish to feel that you dance to the beat of a different drum then you can still do that, but you will find that your inner style will work best and you will be at your most creative at a certain point in the cycle and rhythm of the year. Anarchists or good citizens (is there a difference?) can all have their best feelings and most satisfaction by appreciating the cycles of the earth.

Being Enthusiastic

Nothing succeeds like success. To be successful, you need to be enthusiastic – whether you are cooking a meal, telling a joke or offering help. It sounds trite but a smile and a bit of bustle and activity can make all the difference, both to the energy, and therefore the result, of almost any action. You can even meditate with enthusiasm. A ready smile, and bit of self-propelled motivation, will push a situation along with a momentum over and beyond what you would expect.

You cannot pretend to be enthusiastic, so work at giving yourself an ability to see how things could be improved or made easier. This is the first step to your new enthusiasm. Work at seeing how you could make things more interesting for yourself as well as others.

Practice the art of imagining how you could approach a problem or situation in a new way and try to see how the reaction of the world, to an action of yours, could be the start of a more positive path to follow.

The positive energy that flows into you as a result of an enthusiastic approach cannot be overstated, and needs to be experienced to be believed. Not only do others enjoy enthusiastic people, we also enjoy ourselves more once we're full of passion, inspiration and drive.

You cannot fake enthusiasm, but you can practice at being more vigorous in your attitude to events and imagining how you would feel if you really were full of enthusiasm. You can improve on your lack of enthusiasm for life by being less analytical about an event, show or film and feel its inner vibe that's there if you look for it. By now you may be thinking that this is pointless. By all means, think that, but secretly you will know that this is not the way forward and you are just looking for an excuse not to be more positive. Practice your enthusiastic comments in a mirror and when you try them out, people will respond. Instead of just saying "Hi" when you meet someone, try telling them how nice it is to see them. It will certainly not do any harm.

You can pretend to be enthusiastic, but it is hard to fool people, so make sure your feelings are at least leaning in the positive direction. Equally, if you feel that something is no good then you should be honest and say so! Honesty in a certain situation will make you feel good.

Being Green

This is so obvious that many people lean this way naturally. To be sure of how things work out, we should all try to be greener. The world is a better place with nature being respected and waste eliminated. Although on a personal level being green is fine and dandy, it's also true to say that the least green part of our lives are the giant corporations and unethical businesses that can ruin the earth for the rest of us. Often they are in cahoots with governments, or big money, so it feels as if there is not much that one small person can do. This is where you are wrong. It's the small things that slowly add their weight to the movement towards greenness, moving the world in the right direction despite setbacks. So shoulder to the wheel and remember that Bob Marley sang:

FEELING GOOD

If you are the big tree
We are the small axe
Coming to cut down
Sharpened to cut you down

All you have to do is think green and be green. You are then on the side of righteousness and goodness and this will help make you feel good.

Other good reasons for being green and making yourself feel good are the many opportunities there are for anyone who wants to get involved in signing petitions, writing to politicians and making sure the green agenda, and voice, is heard by anyone who has any power to move the world to a more sustainable and less consuming style.

Feeling good about being green is almost inevitable, as being green has all the fine ethical and moral grounds on its side. When you hear politicians telling you how great GM foods can be, just remember that they are almost all being paid to feel this way, and to reject their ideas is common sense.

To be green you need to recycle and take authorities to task to make sure they get the message. To be green, you must think about helping everyone move toward a greener life. It is no sacrifice to be a bit greener every year. There is not the opportunity to do everything in a sustainable and green manner, but it's the target and the goal to which we need to move to feel good about life on earth.

Bird Watching

A small item in the scheme of things, but we should all try to recognise the birds that live near our homes and find a minute now and then to check them out. If you live in a flat in a city, you may have to visit a park or public space to be able to see a few birds but, wherever you are, there are going to be birds nearby.

They are a resilient type of creature and are great survivors, despite not always receiving favourable treatment from the human race. So check out the local birdlife and if you don't recognise the bird, look it up and find out a little bit about the species. If you travel to work, or go on holiday, there will be different birds along the way to find out about. You don't have to be a professional 'twitcher' to enjoy the sight of a bird, you just need to take an interest, and then you will find you get enjoyment from them – and it is free!

Every year, there are garden-watches organised by

various nature-based charities in which you are invited to spend an hour looking out of your window to see how many birds you can see. It is tricky to spend an hour doing it, but worth it for the information that is shared about how birds are getting along all across the country.

During the winter, you can make yourself feel good by taking a bit of time and a tiny amount of money to feed the birds on your windowsill, in the park or in your garden. Birds will really only feed at your offering if they need it. During the summer, there is an abundance of natural food for them. It's the cold, harsh winters that trouble birds most. Even a few food scraps and an old crust are better than nothing. They are so sweet to watch and your reward is to know that you have helped those birds survive to produce another brood, and give you more birds to watch next year.

You might like to keep a list of the birds you see. It will fill quickly to start with and then it may be months before you see a bird that is not on your list already. When you move to a new home you can start a new list, as you will find that the bird numbers and varieties vary between even quite close areas.

Breathing

When you get in from a day's work, a visit, a school pick up, or whatever, take the time to sit down on a sold kitchen-style chair and take a few slow breaths. Then start with your toes and, whilst thinking of them, take a deep breath in and let it out. Do the same with your ankles and then calves and then knees, till you have covered your whole self. Then take three more slow breaths and get up and carry on as if nothing had happened. You will be surprised by how empowering this is and how simple. It only takes three or four minutes. Do it everyday and feel good.

Become aware of how you breathe and try to breathe deliberately now and then, instead of just surviving by breathing. There are many studies that show how strong breathing sessions can pick you up a bit, and make you feel ready to do more. If you have been breathing hard after a bit of work or a fast walk or run, it's great to think that your blood is being refreshed with all that oxygen. If you find yourself yawning then try taking four or five deep breaths to put yourself back into a more alert state.

When you are walking, your breathing is at a different rate and depth than when you are sleeping or climbing a hill. It's the same old in and out, but with different lengths of time and severity of breath. Once you take an interest in your breath, you will be able to function more efficiently, and with a better degree of consistency, to enable you to continue at whatever you are doing for longer and without becoming tired as quickly as you might expect. Try it!

Mindfulness and breathing are much written about and have become a part of the routine for many practitioners of Eastern philosophies like Buddhism. The essence of the exercise is to detach from everyday concerns and watch yourself taking a breath in and then watch it go out again. The mindfulness of breathing is when you use the breath as an object to concentrate on. By paying close attention to the breath, you become aware of the mind and its jumping about from one thing to another. The simple discipline of studying the breath takes you back to the present moment and what is going on right then. This will give you more clarity.

Clothes and Fashion

Not the obvious fashion statements but, instead, the comfort of wearing clothes that fit and are right for you is something to aim for. It can feel good to be smartly turned out in clean clothes that fit you, but equally it can feel great just lying around in an old tattered sweater and jeans from years ago. It's important that you know what you want from clothes, and not just how you think people expect you to be.

It's not necessary to conform to the kind of uniform-wearing clone that you may feel is necessary to do your job or fit in with fellow workers. At school and as teenagers, people are made to be aware of any straying from what is seen as cool, or the norm, but fortunately as time passes you are able to assert your own style without feeling so persecuted! Feel free to wear something very different to those around you and enjoy the reaction. It does not have to be screamingly

● FEELING GOOD ●

loud or weird, but just a little personal touch to make life more interesting. Even just a very bright pair of socks can liven things up.

Wearing the latest fashion or this year's colour can also make you feel good. A snappy pair of shoes and a sharp outfit can lift your spirits and make you feel on top of the world.

Fashion and your belief in the look you want are all very personal, and individuals will have a different idea of what to wear to make them feel good. It is all about colour, cut and texture and the only way that you are going to get the result you want is by being inventive and thinking about how much it costs, how long it will last and where you are going to be. Many people do not care about how they look beyond a certain point. This is a good thing as the pressure to appear as someone you are not, but maybe want people to think you are, is the oldest trick in the book.

Anti-fashion is a way of expressing your own outlook on life and is also increasingly used as a way of commenting indirectly on the failings of fashion to influence or please yourself. If you live anywhere outside of the West then the whole world of fashion changes as, for the majority of people, it is more about traditional and time-honoured clothing which suits the climate, weather, terrain and vegetation. It is not about look, but instead about practicality and affordability and is probably made by either yourself or a family member. A good fit and comfort are what make you feel good.

Collecting

Not the fancy stuff, but maybe an old bowl or postcard from the Edwardian age. Art is an old book you like or a picture on the wall. Not an antique, but something you like and own because it's more than just a useful thing to you. It may well be useful, but it's not *just* useful – it looks good, too.

Being in touch with well-designed and nicely thought out objects gives you a little bit of art wherever you are. In the world of art galleries and high-end collectible shops there are many beautiful things – buying something for yourself as a treat may be just what you need to put you in a good mood. Collecting something specific, like mirrors or clocks, will give you an insight into the world of art and design that you may not have been interested in before.

See what attracts you and follow your nose. When you have a couple of nice bits of something gorgeous, well made and thought out, you will get more pleasure from them than a boring but smart bit of stuff from Ikea, which may be functional but is rarely artistic.

Stamp collecting is not the most fired-up activity but can give huge feelings of pleasure and satisfaction. Be unconventional in your collecting and make everyday objects your goal. There are a whole lot of different collectibles in the world and one of them will suit you down to the ground, and make you feel good too. Make a list of what you are interested in over a few days or weeks and give some serious thought to the idea of collecting, and consider whether it will drive you crazy, make you a nerd or just a mad, enthusiastic old train set collector. Some people have immense collections of old dolls or lace, or maybe quilts or gloves might take you fancy.

Collecting also includes many associated activities – not just seeking and locating, but also acquiring and then organising. If you are really hooked on your subject then you will move on to cataloguing and maybe displaying your precious things. Looking after and maintaining your collection will also be very interesting and pleasurable.

Computing Skills

It's very handy to have specific skills in computing, like web building, being able to use Photoshop, or understanding design software. These are skills you can acquire through concentration and research, but an evening class or a tutoring course make for a quicker, and more thorough, grounding in the subject. Very useful skills to have, and increasingly a source of satisfaction. Being able to control which direction your keyboard is going to take you is also a basic necessity.

Computer literacy is a very important skill to possess these days. Employers want the people working for them to have all the basic computer skills as their companies become ever more dependent on computers. You will need to be able to learn how to use new software quickly, and practice truly does make perfect.

To really feel good about your internet life, it's not enough to be able to sign up to follow the news, trends,

● *FEELING GOOD* ●

the lives of friends and the latest thoughts on life. It's also crucial to your feeling good that you can set a bit of the pace and involve yourself in the world of communication and design.

You can also earn, if not a living, then certainly a little bit extra as you will find yourself in demand from friends and colleagues once they know you can do something they cannot.

The most common software currently being used for office work is the Microsoft suite of programs for word processing, spreadsheets and presentations. It's important to refresh your skills with these basic programs if they are not well used.

Once you have a few new skills and can do more than just the basics, you will find other skills are easier to acquire. This knowledge base will enable you to feel good about your capabilities and to fit into the newer technologies.

Cooking and Eating In

We should all be able to cook. Cooking is creative and even if there's not much to put in the pan, it's a question of balance and the right herb, spice or packet of sauce to make it more interesting. I've lost you if a ready meal is your idea of feeling good!

Real fresh food can help make you feel good physically and mentally, but processed food – food not straight from nature but straight from a factory – does not have the necessary ingredients to make you function properly. It's possible to live on just jam sandwiches and it may be that this will make you feel okay, but this diet will not enable you to move forward feeling good. There's a difference!

Food is a critical ingredient in how you feel and real food is the thing to go for. Processed food is not easily recognised by the body and the result is that it does not get digested and used properly. We have spent tens of thousands of years eating food that grows, and we are used to it. The new idea of food as something that is made in factories is plain wrong.

If you cannot (or don't) cook then, to start with, set yourself a few simple targets, like scrambled eggs or pasta with a tomato sauce. If you are a reasonable cook already then just work at adding a few more meals to your usual type of cooking, whilst keeping your recipes simple. The things that will make you feel good are going to suggest themselves once you start thinking positively about the result you want. Do some research with friends, relatives, or recipe books and go online to see where you are led with a few keyword searches.

When it come to deciding what to cook, you need to think about the cost of ingredients and the amount of time you are prepared to spend doing some shopping, and then doing the actual business in the kitchen. Some nights you will just want a simple snack to keep you going whilst you are in a dash. Once you get into doing a bit of proper cooking, it stops being a chore and becomes a creative activity in its own right, and can be great fun and very rewarding if you are cooking for someone else too. This will lead to food discussions and maybe you will think of another way to do the same meal again on another occasion.

Dowsing with a Pendulum

This is a simple technique for finding the answer to a puzzle that just may suit you. Not everyone thinks it works, but give it a try – read a couple of articles online or a chapter in a book and see what you think. You don't need any fancy equipment or to spend any money. It's a technique that will put you in touch with a side of yourself you will probably have been ignoring. It's a side that may not need using more than once in a while, but it is an inner ally for you to call on when you need it.

All you really need to start with is a length of thread or string and a small weight, like a key, or a pendant on a chain. Put a question to the pendulum that you know the answer to and see what happens. The best way to establish a successful way forward is to establish 'Yes', 'No' and 'Don't know'. By putting a question to the pendulum like 'Please show me what the 'Yes' reaction is', you will see whether you get a backwards and forwards swing, or an anti-clockwise or clockwise swing. Then you need to find the 'No' and the 'Don't know' responses.

The traditional idea of dowsing would be for the old chap to find water underground for a well or borehole, or to see whether the expectant mother is carrying a boy or a girl. These are simple questions to pose and easy answers to understand. Once you get into less clear cut situations then you need practice in how to pose questions and also how to interpret the answers. This entails practice and research and a bit more reading and intuition on your part.

There are many areas in your life for which you may need to consult your pendulum. The matter of health and medicines are obvious areas for questioning, as are queries about your immediate family and friends. The pendulum does not respond to bad intentions, so you must always think positively about that which you are questing for. Car troubles and practical advice on simple matters are subject for consultation – it is not only metaphysical stuff that you can work with.

Using a simple (or fancy) pendulum will tune you into how the universe works and give you practical insights into what you need to make your life feel good.

Dreaming

A few hours after reading this, you will lose consciousness and slip into a strange twilight world. Where does your mind go during that time known as sleep? And why is it so important that we must spend a third of our lives sleeping?

Recording your dreams and taking an interest in the realm of sleep can show you things that you never knew about your life. Some people remember dreams vividly and some can't remember anything about them. They can be an interesting signpost on your way and are worth thinking about.

If you wake up in the night and are organised, you will have put a notepad and biro by your bed, ready to write down your dream whilst it is still fresh in your mind. Dreams are likely to vanish into thin air unless swiftly recorded, no matter how vivid they may seem.

Some people are able to give an interpretation to

dreams that most of us do not know exist. Dreams are made up of a succession of images and sensations that occur when we are asleep. The purpose of dreams is not fully understood, although they have been a topic of great interest throughout history. The study of dreams is technically known as oneirology.

There are many different interpretations that you can use to understand key parts of your dreams. You can do some research online and even check out a book or two before you start in on the study of dreams. Once you begin thinking about and analysing your dreams, you will quickly realise that dreams are pretty unconnected to your usual worldview and have many aspects that are not just unexpected, but downright weird.

This is all to the good as it shows you that the everyday world that we live in is far more complicated than it appears. Once you have spent a couple of weeks looking at your dreams, you may start to see a pattern emerge. This pattern may be of repeated themes, or storylines and events, or it may be of a certain time or place. The ability to see your dreams close up will make you feel good once you understand that the human mind is not straightforward but highly complicated. This will enable you to start looking at the world from a fresh perspective which will give you those insights into what you need to be a better person.

Driving

Whether it's a pushbike, motorbike, car or a commercial vehicle that you are driving, this can be a great way of feeling free and able to go where you want and not where someone else would like you to go. You don't have to limit your driving to journeys to and from work, shopping or visiting friends and family, you can try just travelling wherever. What happens if you take every third left for thirty minutes? See where you end up.

It's not necessary to drive somewhere in particular – it's the travelling, not the arriving, that for most of our lives is the best bit of any journey. The arriving is either not as imagined, or your expectations remain unfulfilled, and if it does turn out as good as you hoped then you are going to feel good about that. There is no way you are going to be disappointed in this occupation.

We all have an idea about how to drive from an early age. Whether it's pushing a toy car, riding a tricycle

● FEELING GOOD ●

or progressing up to a pedal car and finally a bike – then it's buses and getting lifts from friends and relatives, or the train. But the real freedom of travel is best achieved by actually owning your own transport. This is not practical for everybody as it can depend on where you live, but the joy of the hire car is not to be underestimated. The advantages that a hire care presents can be very liberating.

Whether you are riding a motorbike or driving a car, you immediately know that you could just keep going and soon be in another part of the country, where maybe an adventure or a new sight or friend are to be found. Throughout history, man has enjoyed seeing the world. The other side of the hill is very appealing. Over the hills and far away is an entrancing vision of a better world just around the corner. These are all good reasons to drive down the road.

Not to be ignored are the sheer pleasures of gliding round a nice slow curve or feeling the vibration of the tyres through the frame of the vehicle as road surfaces vary.

If you have driven a lot, you can still get a good feeling from paying attention to all of the aspects of driving that you take for granted. So the next time you head off, be a little more attentive to the idea of driving and sharpen up that good feeling.

Eating Out

Whether you go to a fancy restaurant or a humble café, you can get away from the everyday world and, for a little while, be out of your normal zone. Often the first idea you have is to go to an old favourite place, but trying somewhere new that just opened, or a place that you just heard about is the best answer. When you go out to eat, you should pick something from the menu that you can't make at home, or at least something that is better than you could make yourself. Certainly there is no cooking or washing up to be done, which is always a luxury.

The real good that eating out does is that it relaxes you. It takes you off somewhere interesting where you can watch the waiters and, best of all, you can watch the other people. You can do this openly and discuss them with your fellow diners, or you can check them out of the corner of your eye. Everyone gets pleasure from people-watching and eating out is a great place to do this.

Examining the table layout, the range of dishes and prices, and the way your food looks when it is brought to your table are all most enjoyable. When you are able to just be yourself and not have any worries about the etiquette of eating out, or how much the tip should be, then you are doing it properly.

The mundane responses are the ones to avoid. Do eat with your fingers if the food looks like it will be easier that way. Do not upset the people on the next table with your conversation but, at the same time, do make sure you are not just being polite and feeling a bit dull. Sparkle a bit and chat with your friends or family and make them see that it's alright to relax and not worry. This way, you will feel good having a great time and knowing that all will work out fine. It's not always possible to be at the best table, or the best eatery, but you can have the best time by just enjoying the occasion and the lighting and feel of the place.

You can eat out in the park, on a hill or by a lake. A picnic or barbecue is a fine thing on a decent day – fresh air on the palate makes everything taste better. If you can have a little real fire as well, you will be feeling very good. The wood smoke and sound of sticks burning transports you back to a simpler time. It is not always possible to make the food you want, but there are plenty of simple, wholesome and fun foods that you can put in your hamper or bag to make eating in the countryside well worthwhile.

Exercise and Playing Games

Not everyone likes exercise or playing games. Maybe you got put off at school, or maybe you just aren't a sporty person. You must look instead at what you can do easily to make yourself feel good when you are out and about. If you are leaning this way already, join a local leisure class, or find a friend for a game of tennis or a round of golf.

Joining a football, baseball, cricket or hockey team will be much more of a commitment, depending on the team, but all these activities give your system a huge boost through the release of endorphins and the feel-good effects you get from using your muscles and making your body work hard.

Playing team games is a fine way to spend time with other like-minded people. The after-game break gives you a chance for a chat and to hang out in a zone that's outside of your everyday activities. Maybe you'll go for a drink after a game or training session and then you will have the chance to relax and feel good being part of something.

There are many advantages of playing a sport that raises the activity of your cardiovascular system. You will have a better appetite, you will sleep better and you will also lose a bit of weight and develop a bit of muscle tone, even from just low-level exercise. There are many classes in the keep fit area, from Zumba and Pilates to going to your local gym for a tailored session or a quick work out. You do not need to take out a year's subscription, as nearly all gyms offer a drop-in fee for a set time.

Playing games can be as simple as a crossword or doing Sudoku puzzles. If you did not already know, you will be pleased to hear that playing brain games exercises your cognitive abilities and enhances your brain fitness. So take some time to explore around, play some games, have some fun and improve your brain power in the process. There are jigsaw puzzles and brain teasers that can help. Playing computer games is something very different but can be equally satisfying and very absorbing. Although it is not going to necessarily make you feel bodily good, mentally you may feel great.

Family

Some people are family-minded and some would rather be on their own, but for most of us the family is an item that, one way or another, makes sure we are never alone. The best thing about the family, and its various members, is that there is always someone to talk to and also to talk about. Most families have great strength in the face of adversity. Some people would say that blood is thicker than water and would always put family members ahead of others.

The family you start out with as a child and grow up in as a member is different from the one that you have once you start a family of your own. That is when you will discover how it was for your own parents. The choices and problems that they faced will be shown in a different light that, only now that you are a parent, you come face to face with. They were just as young as you and had to learn on the job, like everyone else.

● FEELING GOOD ●

The older members of the family provide a background of assurance and continuity, with family traditions and jokes getting handed down over the decades. Being part of this will make you feel good. It's your tribe. If there is a bust up or bad feeling between family members, you have to remember that this has always been the case with families and, although regrettable, is something all families live with.

The extended family provide extra interest, with distant cousins and nieces and aunts and uncles. They may seem a bit far away, but they are still family members, and as such easy to say hello to and to fit in with their possibly different lifestyles. Try and stay in touch with as many as you can because this will help everyone feel good and will give you a feeling of a larger family.

The traditional family has been seen as two parents and children, living happily together, and this remains a standard view of life. The reality is that for many, many people, the blended family is how things really are. This makes for all sorts of tensions, and unmentioned secrets, and odd feelings amongst everyone. The path to take to make you feel good about it all is often to bite your lip and hope for the best. The positive steps you can take may be to act as an unofficial mediator and forgiver. This is not an easy role but, when acted on with tact and forbearance, can provide a solution which may make you feel good.

Food

Everyone needs food. Everyone has favourites. Everyone thinks that some ways of cooking are better than others. Everyone has had memorable meals and everyone is interested in food.

Food can make you feel full, overfull, satisfied or just right. Stews warm you up, ginger warms you up. Ice cream cools you down. Chillies and curry burn and then there is Umami – that indefinable but particular savoury fifth taste in addition to sweet, bitter, sour and salty.

Food makes you feel good because it makes you well and healthy. Food makes you feel good because it is sweet and delightful. Food makes you feel good even though you know you should not eat that naughty treat. Food makes you feel good even if the food is not part of your diet!

Processed food, as opposed to real, natural food, is never going to make you feel good over a long period of time – your inner health will be poor and you may become overweight, too. The human race has been eating real food for thousands of years and, as a result, we have adapted to it. If we eat real food, the digestive system knows what to do with it, and how to absorb its nutrients into our bodies.

Processed food is not easy for the system to assimilate as our bodies are not able to recognise it as food. The humble crisp is an early example of processed food, alongside margarine, white bread and sugar. These are all fantastic additions to our lives, but all need treating with care, despite being more or less natural. The packaged ready meal and the pot full of a branded and trademarked foodstuff is the stuff that is processed and, really, is a marketing item rather than food.

The real, feel-good food is simply the old fashioned foods like porridge, salad, vegetables, organic meat, fish, grains and nuts. Olive oil and butter are great for cooking and make food taste better than if you were to use cooking oil.

We can all work out what we need to eat to be healthy, but sometimes we find it expensive. Better to eat a cheap meal of root vegetables and tinned fish than a ready-made, bottom of the range pizza or pie.

Friends

A friend is a person who you know, like, and trust. A friend is someone who you feel close to and whose family and their lives you take an interest in. You may only see each other occasionally, but when you meet you always carry on as if it was only yesterday that you had last seen each other. You can tease and chastise your friends in a way that you could not with anyone else. There are levels of forgiveness and acceptance with friends that you can achieve with no other people. This is what makes you feel good to have friends.

In an ideal world, we would hang out with a great bunch of people and share the same jokes, lifestyle and enjoyment. It does not always work like that, so we make friends, and become acquainted with people we meet as we go. There are childhood friends, school friends, work friends and friends of friends who we hit it off with. The most important point to having friends is to keep in touch with them, and see them if possible. If they move far away, or you go travelling and end up elsewhere, it's crucial to feeling good to make sure they know you want to keep in contact. It's often up to you to make the effort.

Old friends are the tribe you belong to. They are the people who understand many of the ways of the world that you recognise as suiting you, and feeling right. They share some of the same key interests that you have. Whether male or female, the important aspect to feeling good is to know that you belong in a group, gang or crowd whose interests are relevant to you. Many people have a huge number of people they know, but who are not friends. Some people have a very small group of friends and are happy to keep it at that. If you are at all able to find people who you have even just a couple of things in common with, but maybe who make you laugh, or even just know what's good, that's all you need to make yourself feel good.

Friends will come through for you whenever you call them up with a problem. You may think that you should not trouble someone with an issue, but surprise yourself and feel good to find that a friend is always pleased to help and does not feel it is a burden to be part of your life. You would do the same for them if asked. So put yourself in their shoes before you ask, but do ask.

Gardening

Whether you have a house plant or an acre of ground, tending growing leaves and flowers is a thing of joy and all you have to do is put enough time aside to do it. The single house plant on a ledge needs a bit of water and maybe a dead leaf removing from time to time, but will repay you by being interesting and, if it looks healthy and happy, a little bit of feel-good will rub off on you too.

Whatever gardening you are going to do, it's important to realise that growing things contain energy and their own way of life. A vegetable is a short-lived plant, whereas an herb like thyme can live for many years. Some vegetables take a year from seed to the table and some take 12 weeks. In the flower garden, you have short-lived plants that you can grow from seed, or the ones you can get from the garden centre to brighten up a flowerbed, border or planter on the patio. Roses live for a very long time, and their flowers are legendary. Every garden should have at least one.

Being able to join in with the growth of your plants, and their management, will make you feel good. Plants respond to attention and are happy to be pruned, shaped and even dug up and moved to a better position if they do not seem to be thriving where they are. Plants are used to being nibbled by browsing animals.

Planning and thinking about how a plant will give you an enormous sense of pleasure. It can be a thought process that goes on for months, or a spur of the moment impulse to do something to it. Spring is a great time to be outside pottering about and getting things going and even in the autumn, when the sun is low, there are already signs of next year's buds and shoots developing to cheer us up.

Planting shrubs and trees that have a long life is a fine occupation and, if you are able to find space for anything in this line, you will have the interest and satisfaction of seeing growth over a long period of time, or if you have moved to another property you may be able to return years later and see what happened to that Azalea or sapling that you planted.

When you are with your plants and the sun is out, everything you have worked for becomes so very worthwhile and will give you a feeling like no other. Plants fail, they get eaten and plants don't turn out as you expected, but this is all part of the process. It's the ones that work that wipe out any poor growth stories and give you that good feeling.

Genealogy

Take an interest in your forebears. Although at first glance this may seem like a dry, dull occupation, there is nothing like finding out about your roots and what Aunt Gwyneth got up to in 1906.

It is important to know where you come from and what your family has had in their genes, as you share them. Maybe your great grandfather had a profession that's not a million miles away from what you are doing. Your brother, sister or cousin may be a source of support in the project to look back at what went before. It's important to ask your grandparents or aged relatives for any memories they may have or dates that they remember as once they are gone, that information becomes very much harder to gather.

Even if you only draw up the basic family tree of your immediate family, it's a fascinating exercise and, hopefully, over time you may be able to add to the chart you have put together.

There are many online research tools and various software programs that will help you if you become more interested, but that's for when the bug gets you. Once you have your first simple chart then show it to all members of the family and see who can add a date or a half-remembered uncle. The pleasure in putting it together will make you feel good over many years and it may be your grandchildren who pick it up one day and will be grateful that you took the time and care to put it down.

You are going to be doing a bit of research and reading, ringing up old members of the family to glean information and then putting it all down in a practical format. The reason you are doing all of this is not just for you. Although without your interest nothing would get done, you are also putting a family tree together because in years and decades, and even centuries to come, there will be new generations of family members with the same interest. Amongst them, eager searches will be made for the old days, and root-searching will take place to provide a framework within which the family exists. The knowledge that you are putting together will not only fascinate you and make you feel good, but will also make future family members feel good about their history and forebears.

Health

It may seem obvious that part of feeling good is to be, and to stay, healthy. But health is not just about being fit. You can suffer from a bad back or a sore ankle, or a variety of life changing afflictions, and yet still be classed as healthy. So, health is not just being able to run a marathon, or being an ideal weight, or feeling that you will live forever. It's also about an acceptance that being human means that you will have a niggle here and an itch there for most of your life.

Catching a cold does not make you unhealthy and, as a result of the cold, your immune system will be strengthened against future illness – there is a heath benefit over time. The secret to feeling good about your health is not to have unrealistic expectations about how you are going to be.

To feel good about your inner health, you must make sure that you are up to a bit of exercise, even if it's just walking a mile. It's the key to having the confidence that you could dash up the stairs in an emergency, or run for that train or bus without feeling like you are going to keel over from the effort. The same is true with your reaction to any illness or damage. If you are fairly well fed, and not unfit, then your recovery from a setback will be that much quicker and more rounded.

To ensure your health is good, and that therefore you feel good, it is essential to be aware of your fitness levels and your diet, as well as to make sure you are getting enough sleep and not taking your body for granted. You need to top up your natural health with whatever seems to you to be required. Only you know how you really feel, and so only you can have the opportunity to make sure that you stay healthy, feeling as good as possible.

Garlic, olive oil and the Mediterranean diet seems a sound basis to build your health on, along with a glass of red wine now and then. Drink fresh water, not canned or fizzy drinks, and try not to use any man-made sweeteners which seem implicated in many heath issues. Check any food supplements you are taking have no queries against them and make sure that you are eating as many different things as possible to ensure a good intake of trace minerals.

Hobbies

Hobbies are not just about stamp collecting or traditional pastimes. A hobby could be described as an activity, interest, or enthusiasm that is undertaken for pleasure or relaxation, usually during one's free time.

The best sort of hobby is not one that you feel forced into by circumstance, but one that suits your age and spare time and that you feel passionate about. Make sure that whatever you do is for you and you alone. Other people's opinions are just that, opinions, and they should be ignored!

Hobbies are not always definable, but have a role to play in keeping you feeling good by giving you contact with a pleasure on a regular basis. Work out what you need and see whether you can find time to carry out the essential part of a hobby, which is concentrating on something interesting and letting the everyday world slip away for a little while.

Sometimes a hobby can develop into a business or a way of making a bit of extra money. Some hobbies enable you to meet up with other people with the same interests. Hobbies are mainly enjoyed due to the need to spend time doing something that takes us away from the stresses of life – not something that will make you stressed.

The very best hobbies are the ones that you kind of fall into through a set of circumstances, rather than a planned agenda to do something. This is ideal and should not be fought, or resisted, but encouraged to flower and develop and carry you along with the tide of information, and interest, that it will generate.

There are lists of hobbies that you can consult if you feel that you must do something in your life other than watching TV or spend hours staring at a screen. Whether it be model making, or fashioning old time quilts, you will want to find something that can absorb you over long periods. You may only put in an hour now and then, but it is something that you can pick up and carry on with whenever there is an opportunity. If your life feels empty and drab, this will help make you feel good.

Holidays

There is a constant pressure to take a holiday and the right break, vacation or long weekend is something of value. For some people, this can mean travelling the world on a gap year, and for others it's a mini-break in an economy hotel, or just a day at the beach or shopping. It's not what you do, it's the fact that you are doing something to get out of the everyday round that, without you realising, is holding you captive. As soon as you get away, you get a different view of what you are, what you do and are given a chance to do something different.

Travel broadens the mind because you get to see other things, other people, and different lifestyles and ways of feeling good. So, make sure to find any chance of getting away from the everyday whenever you can. Ideally this would be a luxury visit but very often, it's the ordinary stay that you forget and the intensity of the out of the ordinary that works best. If you spend your holiday cosseted in a sumptuous environment, you may find that the only thing that stands out in your memory is the fact that it was a luxury break, rather than the details of an ordinary place that enabled you to have more memorable experiences that will stay with you.

When it is that you are able to have a holiday depends on your work, where you go depends on a variety of factors, who you go with is a personal choice, how much you spend is dictated to you by circumstance. The one thing you should really concentrate on to make yourself feel good is to at least make it a two week stay, visit or holiday. Less than this and you will find that by the time you have slipped down into a nice easy relaxed feeling, it's time to wind yourself back up to go home. A two-week time out gives you time to slip deeply into relaxed mode for several long days and over a year that feeling will stay with you. This will enable you to tap into deep sources of energy, health and strength-building that will ensure you will be able to cruise through the hard work ahead of you.

Lifestyle

This is more about how you feel you can fit into the world, and how you can make the most of what you have. Lifestyle is not about being rich and carefree. Lifestyle is about how you keep yourself feeling good by doing the right things for yourself. This may well be by trying to look wealthier than you are and striving to live like a rich person when you have no money. This approach won't make you feel good all the time.

What will make you feel good is enjoying what you have and making the most of it. Living cheaply and organically in a green way will make you feel better if it's done in a positive way, and not just because you feel you should. You must want what it gives you. Better free than a slave!

Many people feel that they do not have a lifestyle, but are carrying on as they like just because that's how they are. However, to other people looking at those same lives, they would describe them as having a specific lifestyle. This is interesting because it means that nobody really knows how they are perceived by the public, but equally they have an opinion on the public they meet.

It would therefore be pointless to try and guess how you are seen. The smart move is to do what you feel is right for you. This may be to keep up an appearance, but this is not going to make you happy even if it does tick some boxes on your imaginary to-do chart. Your needs are to keep yourself feeling happy by being who you want to be, and doing what you want to do. The strength required to be yourself is the strength to overcome the feeling that you must conform. It is the issue that you need to resolve in order to be yourself, and to be able to ignore the urge to fit in with other peoples' ideas of how you should live your life.

Lifestyle choices are not simple and they will depend on where you live. Your lifestyle in a town will be different from the lifestyle you might have if you lived in the country.

Medication

In the West, medication has become very common for a variety of ailments and afflictions and has become a crutch for the insecure and a prop for the unwell. In the old days in China, you only paid the doctor when you were well.

If you are on medication, there is the old problem of side-effects and the trade-off between treating one condition and possibly acquiring another. The secret is to find the right balance that makes you feel good. Just because the advised treatment is supposed to make you feel good does not mean that this is what will happen.

You need to take control of the situation and find the balance that works. There are many ways to feeling good and only you know the ones that will work for you. Be prepared to look at alternatives, do research and ask friends and fellow sufferers for advice and insight. There are plenty of chances to find information online but remember to make up your own mind, as even the world's greatest experts are not always right.

Medication can be a fantastic help in your life. However, there are many stories where medication has either just masked a condition that could have been treated differently or has caused other problems. Combining two or more medications can cause more problems than they solve – thus requiring more medication.

Medication is a route that, for many doctors, provides an easier answer than looking at other, simpler ways to treat conditions. So, whilst not wanting to lose trust in your doctor, it is important to question a doctor's decisions and research the possible alternatives.

Feel free to discuss these matters with your friends and colleagues and do online research. Some simple exercises can be better for you than taking medication. Drinking a litre of water may cure your headache better than a couple of aspirin.

Meditation

Meditation is a well-known activity, but in reality is not easily started as a practice. You can stare out of the window, you can daydream, you can snooze, you can let time drift by in various ways, but meditation requires determination and desire. There are many classical forms of meditation and there is no agreement as to which form is more useful, or the best. The one thing that everyone involved agrees on seems to be that you will gain the ability to stay calm, and feel good, whatever happens.

Initially, whichever form of meditation you settle on is not important, as once you start to settle into a few minutes of careful cooling down and sitting quietly, you will be led to a form of meditation that suits you best at the time in your life that you have started out. Read articles, books and even talk to people to gain clarity over what you need to do to find the style and

● FEELING GOOD ●

practice that suits you best. Only you will know this, so be brave and go with that which appeals to you rather than that which either you feel you should do, or that which someone else feels you should do.

Meditation refers to many practices that each include techniques designed to enhance and help your relaxation, to build internal energy or life force and to help you to be more compassionate and patient as well as increasing your generosity of soul, love and forgiveness.

Meditation has been practiced for at least two thousand years as part of numerous religious traditions and beliefs. Meditation often involves the effort to self-regulate the mind. It can be used to ease your mind and help with some health issues, such as high blood pressure, depression and anxiety.

If you decide to include meditation in your life, you do not need a guru or mentor, but you might find it handy to have a chat with someone already doing it, or watch an instructional clip online, to give you a few insights into the best way to start out. All you need to start feeling good with your new practice is something to sit on, comfy clothes and a fairly quiet room or space.

Music

You may not play an instrument, but you can enjoy listening to music. The music that's going to make you feel good is the music that works for you. The only definition of good music is music that you personally like. The arguments will always rage on about this music being better than that, or the other having a better beat or superior lyrics, but what you want to hear at any given time will not be the same as someone else. Make sure you listen to what you like.

Drumming and just beating a stick on a rock are how most people believe music started out in prehistory and, to this day, it is very pleasant to do just that. When no one is around, you might like to have a go at getting a rhythm and a beat going by drumming on the back of a chair or tabletop.

Classical music is a whole world into which some people step and enjoy. A lot of the music from the days of European courts and their sponsors is well known and much enjoyed, but most of it has fallen by the wayside as it really is hard to empathise with.

Old jazz and blues from the 1920s and 1930s formed the roots of modern music. There are some great recordings available from those days. Every era since has thrown up a certain style and type of music, from jazz to hip hop. If you have never taken the time and effort to listen to styles that are different to the ones you grew up with, then you have missed out on a major opportunity to feel good.

If you play an instrument then maybe you would like to get together with another musician or two and see whether it might be fun to make a little music together. If you have never had a chance to learn to play an instrument then you could think about taking lessons, or teaching yourself to play something like the harmonica.

Listening to live music is very different from that which comes through your headphones. The immediacy and vibration of a real instrument being played close by is like nothing else to set the pulse racing. Whether it's a full classical orchestra or just a band in the local nightspot, you have got to get out and listen for yourself. Live music is just about guaranteed to make you feel good.

Optimism

'Always look on the bright side of life' is a good guide to positive living. Seeing the glass half full rather than half empty is a way of seeing the world in a better light. It's not always possible to be cheery and upbeat about the life we live, but it's still true to say that if you want to feel good then being an optimist is a great start.

There are of course natural pessimists – those who enjoy seeing the gloomy side – and if this makes them feel good then there's a bit of an intuitive leap to be made about feeling good. Not all is simple. It is not all black and gloomy and even though you may quite like it to be that way, there is no reason not to try a little positivity to see what happens. With an optimistic outlook, you are better able to cope with tricky situations.

It may not seem easy, or natural, to be a glass half full type of person, but all it really requires is a modicum of effort, and not much time, to generate a more relaxed outlook on life and life events. The trick is to work at it over a period of months and always seek out the positive and more uplifting aspects to a situation that, in the past, you would not have bothered with. If, of course, it turns out that the problem was hopeless, this does not negate the approach you have made of trying to make it better!

The great advantage of attempting to see the good in people and in what is happening is that there is a positive feedback to the situation. This positive feedback engenders better responses from the people, and situations, that you are involved with. This is because you will be seen as someone who can benefit others and promote good vibes in all things associated with you. You will find people are more wiling to forgive mistakes, and to try and help, with the positive spin you are putting on everything.

Pets

Owning a pet is well known to lessen stressful feelings in addition to providing you with a companion. The type of pet you have is going to make a big difference. Owning a stick insect or lizard is not the same as a friendly dog or purring cat, but it's what appeals to you that counts, so don't be put off getting an unusual pet just because other people think it might not work out. Cats and dogs are pets all over the world because of their ability to relate to, and be with, their human tribe. Dogs are particularly good at inserting themselves into your life and making themselves feel needed! Going away on holiday or just for the day is always tricky if you have a pet, but the responsibility of pet owning is part of the experience. Going on holiday with a pet can also be a great way to reinvent your relationship, as new situations arise when away from home which lead to new solutions which, when you get back home, can be put into effect.

FEELING GOOD

The feel-good factor of your relationship with your pet is the main reason for having a pet, unless you feel that looking after an abandoned animal is an act of humanity that you cannot deny. This sort of pet owning is difficult to begin with, but will give you an immense reward once you have surmounted the problems that often occur with animals that have been abandoned, or were unwanted. Do pick your companion with care as it's no use trying to change your life around to fit in with an animal that cannot fit in with you.

If you feel that an attack dog, or a big fierce dog, is going to provide you with a degree of protection, it is probably true. On the flip side, it may be that it is not going to make you feel good as well. The breed of animal is an important aspect to your choice and one that must be given consideration.

All animals need time and care, but most are able to give something back to earn their feed. The most aloof cat has its moments of friendly behaviour to endear them to you.

Photography

You only need a basic mobile phone to own a camera. The quality may be a little low, but much enjoyment can be had taking pictures of friends and family. Take it a step further and get a camera with 10+ megapixels and you now have something that can challenge the very best. The top-end cameras are not for the casual snapper, and run into serious money.

Before the digital age you needed real film, there was no useful autofocus and taking a photograph was much more serious a business. Firstly because of the procedure of focus, aperture and speed of shutter, and then there was the cost of the film and developing. Much enjoyment can still be had with this type of equipment, but it really is only for the dedicated craftsperson.

Once you have the pictures you like, the enjoyment lies in working with them in a software programme that allows you to improve colour, crop and otherwise alter.

● FEELING GOOD ●

Photoshop is the best known, but there are a multitude of other choices that you may find more suited to you.

When you are out and about with your camera, you need to look around for a shot of sufficient interest and the more you look, the harder it can be. There are always easy shots, like of sunsets or snow or more arty shots. But look beyond the immediate and see if you can find an everyday something which, taken from an unusual angle, or into the sun, or with a shadow, can be transformed into a wholly different thing.

Taking pictures of people is a bit tricky as it is literally in your (their) face. The reward for taking pictures of people, though, is that they are what everyone wants to see – the favourite photo of a tree in the mist just does not grab the attention like a picture of your friend's screwed up face after eating a bite of lemon. It does take a certain amount of courage to take pictures of people as, if you know them, they will complain that their hair is wrong, while taking pictures of strangers is just that. Once you have got into the habit of taking pictures of people, the best bit is looking at them later on, maybe years later. The feel-good factor in photography is that you are creating something for yourself which you can also share.

Poetry

Writing poetry is good for the soul. There's a wide variety of poetry, from simple rhyming lines, through to limericks and song lyrics. There's long, rambling prose that sits in pentameters and hexameters, there's love poems and Japanese Haiku and then, of course, there is the poetry that you want to write. It may be a mix of different styles, it could be conventional, or it could be wild and experimental. The only way to find out what you like to write is to start writing.

All you need is a pencil, or pen, and a bit of paper. You can type poetry in Word, but its not quite so flexible as a hand tool and scrap of paper.

You will quickly find that your first idea is probably the best because, as you become more self-conscious about what you are writing, it may go downhill. If you keep going, it will then become more like the idea you had to start with. It's a process that involves trial and error and a bit of staring into space wondering what to write next and if it sounds silly.

There is such a huge body of work that has already been produced, over many thousands of years. Most ideas have been tried out already, so you may not be looking to produce unique work. You might look instead to reinterpret popular moods and themes, and relive the simplest of ideas, as it's your own voyage of discovery. The delight and wellbeing you can obtain from a couple of well-written lines will certainly make you feel good. You are writing for yourself and if you want to show your work to others, then that is a step for you to decide to take.

When you first sit down to write a poem or a few lines of prose, try to let your mind come up with a random subject and just start writing and see where you go. You may want to try a classic four-liner, or a ditty with no deep meaning. There is of course also the chance to do something very obscure and deep, hundreds of lines long. Writing poetry needs a bit of practice and you will find that rhyming is not as easy as you may imagine. Check out some of the great poets and see how they resolved these issues.

Random Acts of Kindness

There is no finer thing in life than to help other people. Just randomly being nice to someone, or helping them in some small matter, is not expensive, takes little energy and can be done almost anywhere at any time. It does require you to be willing to put yourself in a position of improving the world. This is not hard. This is not rocket science. At its simplest, it could be picking up something that someone has dropped or helping a person with a door. It is what used to be called politeness, or chivalry, or just neighbourly.

So, if you go out with a positive attitude and a wish to make someone's day a little better then you could set yourself a target to do one good deed a day. You could do one good deed every week. Ideally, you would just perform a random act of kindness now and then, when the moment is there. If you are going to wait for the perfect opportunity to appear, you may be in for a long wait. The best thing to do is keep your eyes open and be alert to possibilities.

The idea of practicing random kindness, and senseless acts of beauty, is a selfless act performed by someone wishing to either assist or cheer someone else up. As such it will make you feel good, too. You may never know the effect that your action has on someone else's situation, or outlook on life. It almost certainly will not be bad, however!

You could try just giving someone a flower or, if you know them well, a hug can be good. A smile is friendly and a small moment of your life may unlock a whole new approach in your mind.

When a random act of kindness is carried out, your brain will associate this with happiness and trust. The best thing is the feel-good endorphins that are released in the people involved. Happiness is also contagious and so, if you're happy and you associate with another person, their happiness increases. When that person connects with another person then their happiness increases too. It a win-win situation, so do go out and see if you can spot an opportunity to make this happen.

Reading

Reading a newspaper or an advertisement is not always going to make you feel good. Reading a magazine, whilst it may hold your attention, is so often a lifestyle thing. Reading a book or short story, or an essay, or a vivid piece of prose has much more chance of making you feel good. The classic short story is one that can be read in one go and can be filler for a train journey, or used to settle you down before you go to sleep – it will always be popular. There are books on how to live your life, or how to mend a computer or drive a car, or a million instructional actions to make life easier.

Books are lively things and burst with ideas and possibilities. A good long book will give pleasure over many days and can give you something continuous, and fascinating, to follow. A real story is not hard to find and, whether it's a classic Dickens or one of the

● FEELING GOOD ●

numerous authors who are household names, there's always a book waiting to be read.

So sit yourself down with a nice light and a good cup of tea or lemonade and relax into a book. You can set the pace and decide when to stop and start, when to stare into space and when to break for a bite. It's not like watching a film or a documentary – you are the boss and can decide the timing. It may feel old-fashioned and quiet, just sitting there reading, but persevere and you will come to appreciate the space it gives you, and the relaxation you can achieve by not doing anything but being totally absorbed.

While you are reading, apart from being enthralled by the story, you may also notice the style the writer has and how the narrative or plot keeps going along. A lot of thought has gone into most books, and a study of the book that you are reading is always worth a bit of time. It enhances the book and helps you to feel involved.

Reading out loud to an elderly relative or a young child is fantastic and you will not regret a minute of time spent on this simple activity. With children, you need to find a story that is either simple or lightly written. Treasure Island is too long for young children, but your elderly relative who is not well would certainly enjoy it and you will feel very good with an attentive audience.

Running

Anyone can run. You may feel embarrassed to be seen running, you may not look like an international athlete, but just a slow jog when no-one is looking, or a trot around the park, are the sort of easy things you could try to start with. You can just break into a jog for a few steps now and then, as if running for a bus. If you live in the country you can usually find a quiet spot, while in the city an early morning outing might be possible.

The act of running, and therefore breathing harder, are well known for their positive effects on your whole system. Not just at the time, either, but over the next 24 hours too. You may be stiff and sore for a couple of days after your first run. This is a good thing and shows that you can do it, but should not overdo it! Just do a bit when you feel its right and slowly build up, or just keep it at an occasional trot – it is all about changing yourself into a more able and efficient person.

● FEELING GOOD ●

When you run, it is important to breathe properly and steadily. It should come automatically, but unless you are used to it, breathing is more complicated and will need some thought. The same goes for thinking as you run – it's a good time to let your subconscious take over and to let random thoughts and ideas tick over. It is also a good time to work out any frustrations or problems in your life, which can often come to seem less pressing as a result.

You will need a pair of trainers and loose clothing and, if you get over heated, just take off the top layer of your clothing. It is handy to carry a bottle of water to drink along the way. This can also be poured over your head if you need to cool down, which always feels good.

Running past your fellows, head held high, is one of the great natural highs to be gained from running. You feel healthy, fit and in control. But do remember that roads have traffic, so be ready to alter your pace, and run on the spot while you wait for the cars to go by.

Before you start running, remember to do a few basic stretches and walk for a couple of minutes before you break into a run, to get your muscles moving. This will make sure you feel good during your run.

Singing

It is not always a wonderful day coming your way, and it's not always a sad song. Singing in the shower or bath is a nice, private way to show yourself that all is not lost. Singing as you drive the car is a popular expression of gladness, as you will notice if you study your fellow drivers. A car is a private space, and no one else can hear you.

Singing exercises the lungs and makes you think about what, and how, you sing. Some of us have great, easy voices that work without effort. Some of us cannot sing in tune. It does not matter – all you have to do is give it a quiet breathy song no-one can hear, or just get on with it and not care who hears. There's always a chance that a friend, family member or partner will complain, but that is not the end of the world.

'Singing in the Rain' is a fine example of how singing can augment a good feeling and give you a chance to celebrate that feeling. Not all singing is celebratory – sometimes you can just sing along to the radio or the music in your earphones. The joy of singing is that there are so many different types of singing styles, all the way from opera to rap.

Your singing can be formal or easy, written down or made up. You can sing for fun, comfort or profit. To get good at singing may require time, instruction and some practice. You may feel that it's not that important in your life, and therefore that it requires no more than just suddenly bursting into a song. Whistling is another fine way to express yourself and fulfil that inner urge to be creative with your breath.

Singing in a band, choir or a folk club is another option that could be the avenue to get you going. There are a capella clubs and there are simple occasions when you can sing, maybe in a church as a member of the congregation. You could practice a song with your partner or friend to surprise your acquaintances. Many years ago, before any technology existed, an evening around the piano, with duets and the singing of traditional songs, was the standard way to pass the time.

Sleep

Without good sleep, life can seem harder. We don't all need those eight hours, but it is nice to get a good night's sleep. Up until the industrial revolution, everyone would have had an early night and, as research tells us, may have had two separate sleeps having been up for a couple of hours in the night. Very often, those sleepless nights are an echo of how we lived before electricity.

There is no point lying awake wondering if you will ever get back to sleep. There are a couple of good techniques for getting you back to sleep if you're still awake after an hour or so. The first is to take 14 very deep breaths in and out, as fully as you can. This should be done slowly and deliberately. The second is to start with your toes and tell them to relax, and then work all the way up through your body to your hair, telling each part of your anatomy to go to sleep.

● FEELING GOOD ●

A good sleep aids healing and restores the inner being. You need a decent bed and a good mattress with a choice of duvet and blankets, so that whether it's summer or winter, you will have the right covering. A lot of people just put up with whatever they happen to have already but, with sleep taking up such a large part of our lives, it is worth spending some time analysing the missing ingredients in your sleeping arrangements and putting them right.

Whether it is something simple like a new pillow or sheet, or a nice new duvet, the cost is not high enough to stop you getting the balance right. The mattress is the costliest item and needs to be invested in to make your life better. Treat the choice seriously, and spend some time looking for the type of mattress that will keep you comfortable, even if you have to save up for it. Once you are sleeping better, you will wish you had done it earlier.

Some of us of us try to cut down on sleep. There are so many things that seem more interesting or important than an early night, but just as exercise and good food are essential for feeling good, so is sleep. The type of sleep you're getting directly affects the quality of being awake, including your mental agility, creativity and vitality. There is nothing that delivers as many benefits, and helps make you feel good so easily, as a good night's sleep!

Spirituality

You don't have to belong to a church or a movement or organisation to have a spiritual life. Christians, Buddhists, Muslims, or any other of the well known belief systems don't have a lock on spirituality. There are so many ways of feeling at one with, or at least part of, the universe and the life and energy of the place you are in.

Personal well-being and development and the idea of spiritual experience are all a part of a worldview that can make you feel good. Throughout most of Europe in the middle-ages, the idea of spirituality was mainly governed by what your priest said. The ancient Greeks and Egyptians had a very different view of the world and how a human could fit into the spiritual dimension.

In the modern world, it has become accepted by many people that a looser definition is required to enable you to take control of your understanding of the way the world works. Spiritual life has become a matter of personal interpretation – that which makes you feel good may be a view you hold that others don't. This is to be encouraged and you must have the chance, and also the belief, to realise that the world is as you see it – and not just as you are told it is. The opportunity to mould a view of life and the universe that suits you will make you feel good. Do not be deterred from developing your own opinions and views.

Spirituality means something different to everyone. For some, it's about going to a church, synagogue, or mosque. For others, it's very personal. Some people feel in touch with their spiritual side through quiet prayer, yoga, meditation or even just walking.

Recent research finds that most spiritual sceptics cannot avoid the sense that there is something greater out there. As we process experiences, we look for patterns and then seek meaning in these patterns. We can't help but ask what is going on – the impulse seems to be part of how our minds work. To make yourself feel good about your relationship with the Universe, you can spend some time thinking about these things.

Star Gazing

On every clear night, there is a fantastic free show just outside your door, which many people never look up to see. In a big city or town, the streetlights may well drown out all but the moon and a couple of the brightest stars, but if you are living anywhere near the countryside then the stars are there for your pleasure. You may know the big dipper, or the Pole Star, but most people could not even find Venus on a clear night.

Looking at the stars on a fine summer evening is the most romantic and satisfying occupation. You don't need a telescope or binoculars to start with. All you might like to have is a star map to refer to whilst you learn the names of the major constellations.

So, here's a nice little project for you. Do a little research and see if you can spot Pegasus or The Pleiades. Then, try and add one celestial feature every month. This will mean that there is always something to look out for that you can recognise in the night sky and that you can take an interest in.

The moon is a fine sight and following the phases of the moon, and knowing without even looking whether the moon is waxing or waning, will help put you in touch with the rhythms of the world and your life. The moon has a huge influence on the way we feel and what we do. Very often, you will find that your biorhythms can be judged by where the moon is. You may find that you are at your best when there is no moon, or at the start of the new moon cycle. It will take a while to work this out as we are all different. Once you know when you are feeling good, it is possible to set tasks to fit in with this state. When you are feeling at a low ebb you can relax, secure in the knowledge that it does not matter, as you will be able to catch up when your positive feelings coincide with the lunar phase that indicates you are on top of the world.

Amateur astronomers regularly surprise scientists by finding objects that have been missed. This has been true for comets and meteors as well as larger discoveries like supernovae, very much further away. It's a classic calling: going back to the dawn of time, when the fire at night and the starry skies were a big part of peoples' lives.

During the winter months, the cold nights can give very bright, clear and star-filled skies but it can force you to hurry back in to warm up. When you can look up at the sky and know what you are looking at, you will feel great satisfaction and you will also be able to help others name a few constellations and key stars.

Supporting a Team

This may sound a little like old-school style thinking, but the team you support could be a top class football team or it could be a village side. Maybe skittles or the local cricket club take your interest. There are a multitude of other teams you could take an interest in, from women's archery to ice hockey.

At school, we generally had little choice in what the organised activity of the season was. Everyone having to be a winner and everyone being made to participate may be a memory that you would rather forget about. Supporting a team skips around this, and gives you the chance to be part of something bigger than just yourself.

You could take an interest in all sorts of competitive games involving teams that are broadcast on television – some large and some tiny, all the way from Strictly Come Dancing to University Challenge. It is almost impossible not to feel affection and a certain hope that a particular side you take an interest in will come out on top.

The hunting pack and tribal, ancestral memories dictate how we view the world. It's instructional to use the opportunity of following a team for a day, or over many years, to give you a sense of feeling good – although it can be tinged with the disappointment of doing poorly. But, even in defeat, there are things to take forward to the next occasion when your support and interest in another situation will revive. So, it's not just about the winning or losing, it is also the taking part and not being shy about putting your own doubts to one side and feeling partisan.

Teams that everyone is aware of are great to follow and take an interest in, but tiny local teams are not without their charm and will contain a selection of interesting characters and personalities. Underdogs are easy to like, as are the very talented. Teams with a lot of skill or none whatsoever are strangely likeable. The reasons don't need to be valid or even last beyond the end of the game, but that sense of belonging makes contests seem important.

Travel

This is a great opportunity to make yourself feel good. A lot of our travelling is just to work, or visiting friends. These routine, everyday sort of journeys may sometimes involve an interesting event, but are usually entirely forgettable or just a chore.

Going away on more than just a holiday will make you feel especially good. Planning for a trip, as well as looking forward and imagining how it's going to work out and what you will need to take with you, are all very much a part of the journey. You will have to decide where you are going and how you are going to get there. You might do some online research. You'll think about how much it will cost and the most economic way of doing it. You will have to decide on travelling companions and how it will work out – maybe you are going with a long-time partner, or maybe you're going alone. What clothes you will need and whether you

● FEELING GOOD ●

need vaccinations or a visa are important points to consider. These are all part of the multitude of things you'll need to think about, and are a very big part of the interest and pleasure to be found in travelling.

Whether you are going for a week, a month or many months, there is an element of luck and chance as to who you will meet along the way and how your perceptions of the world will change. The old saying that travel broadens the mind is totally true and provides a very good reason to travel in the first place

Another good aspect of travelling is that, when you return, you can look back on what happened and what went wrong and remember just how interesting it all was. Maybe you have photos to look at, a purchased souvenir, or just a nice stone that you picked up by the road or from a stream bed. This will give you a topic of conversation and memories that you can revisit over the years. Travelling is more intense, and vivid, than most of your everyday life and is a must to make you feel good.

Using a Tarot Pack

Using a Tarot pack may feel like a step into the unknown, but for thousands of years they have been used to offer guidance and comfort from their use as divination aids. The ability to read a set of circumstances which, when delivered by a force that comes from the heart of being, opens a door to a world of choice and a path of positive action, cannot be ignored. Being able to sidestep issues down the line and to be forewarned of problems is a great helper on your path to feeling good.

The older styles of divination include Runes and the I Ching. There are no set rules for which style or type of tarot will work best for you. A little research and you will find you are drawn to one of the many types of tools there are. They represent a triumph of man's intuitive knowledge that all is not as it seems. It is very important to grasp a chance to feel good about your fate and path through life and to be able to see

● FEELING GOOD ●

that a simple technique can have a great force for good.

There are plenty of people who will say it's a load of old tosh, and if you are one of them then it's just not for you. However it is more than likely that, if you are reading this, you are interested.

Once you have your chosen pack and have spent a little time understanding it and the process required, you will need to look after it and keep it somewhere safe. Be aware that a little respect is called for to get the best result. One of the most difficult things about reading Tarot cards is keeping an open and clear mind and staying objective. You will soon pick up the basics and become proficient

Finding out how to read Tarot cards takes a combination of knowledge and intuition that will take you a little while to develop. Once you have become proficient, you may feel like going a step further and offer to do readings for other people. The help you can offer will make you feel good.

Walking

Walking is free and presents one of the best ways to get more active and feel healthier. It's not famous as a form of exercise, but walking is ideal for everyone. Regular walking has been shown to reduce the risk of chronic illnesses. Shoes are all you really need, and any shoes or trainers that are comfy, and provide support, will do. However, if you decide to do walking more often and to go further, then a good pair of walking shoes are a must. After your first pair has worn out and you have got used to your new ones, you will get extra pleasure from being unaware that your shoes are even there, which is the sign of a good walking shoe

Start off leisurely and try to build up your walking time and speed over a couple of weeks. To feel good from walking, you need to go at a moderate-intensity aerobic rate once you are a little fitter. In other words, it needs to be faster than a stroll.

If, to begin with, you can only walk fast for a couple of minutes, that's fine. Don't overdo it on your first day. Begin your walking slowly and then increase your pace. After a few minutes, if you're ready, try walking a bit faster still. Near the end of your walk, gradually slow down your pace.

When you're walking to the shops or part of your journey to work, try to make every step count. The best way to walk more is to make walking a routine. Think of some ways to include walking in your daily life. You don't have to travel to the country to find a good walk – urban spaces offer many interesting walks, including parks and riverside paths. Walking in a group is a great way to start more serious walking, make new friends and stay motivated.

Whilst you are walking is a great time to let the brain tick over about many ideas that may have been troubling or interesting you. The subconscious act of steady walking is a pleasure in itself, just being able to look around at the passing scenery, whether it's in a town or the country, is part of the beneficial side to walking. You can easily overlook the benefits, as it's not just about getting or keeping physically fit – the exercise you get from walking not only prevents depression, but can also treat it. The endorphins released when completing this physical activity can immediately lift your mood, along with improving your ability to sleep. Another good thing about exercise like this is that it gives you the opportunity to remove yourself from technology.

Watching Old Movies

Now, here's an easy way of feeling good. There's nothing like watching an old-time movie to generate good feelings. The brand new movie, the one that gives you a buzz and is the latest thing, is the one that everyone wants to see, but the new releases are generally set in the context of now. An old movie (and not just last year's, but one from the distant past) has the advantage of being set in a known history. There is nothing unexpected in the general context, as you know the world carried on in a certain way after the era of the film. You know that everything turned out alright.

For the strongest historical and cultural impact, older movies are well worth watching. They are superb time capsules, capturing the look and music of an earlier time. Before the introduction of film, it was almost impossible to have a realistic idea of what living in an older time period was like. With any film, you can look back into periods of time that have long since passed.

A lot of older movies have better stories and plots. In the earlier age of film, there was no CGI or studio-made special effects – it was all done in a more realistic and convincing way. A great many older movies rely on clever scripts, plot twists, talented actors and an interesting story rather than the blockbuster look. So, make sure you really check out the hats and shoes and styles that people went for in the past. Its surprising how little has changed and yet how different the whole look and feel of an old film can be.

The very early films were black and white and whether it is Laurel and Hardy, Charlie Chaplin or the Marx Brothers, the whole genre seems to be aimed at tickling the audience's sense of humour. Well worth watching a few to make you feel good.

Cowboy films were all the rage in the fifties as an antidote to the war. Many are still excellent at bringing to life a romanticised way of living that is still revered, although long gone. Find a genre that intrigues you and watch as many as you can to get in the mood of the time and place. Highly recommended are the noir films with Bogart and Bacall.

Work and Jobs

You have to earn a living and probably are not able to choose exactly the job you end up doing. The secret of making a job enjoyable and feeling good about what you do can be achieved by turning off all of your inner soul instincts and just doing a job like a drudge, with no more effort involved than is necessary to avoid being fired.

You could, however, approach the same job in a different way – you could force yourself to be enthusiastic and seek the best way to do everything. Some people might think that they were kidding themselves with this approach and the answer may lie elsewhere. The alternatives are to not take a job you aren't wild about, to do no job, or to hope something will turn up that will make life worthwhile. The choice is yours. One way to feel good at work that you are not enjoying is to use it as a means to an end and not the end itself.

Some jobs are great and a lot may depend on the people you work with, not what you have to do. Some jobs are great full stop!

If you aren't happy in a traditional job role, you could consider becoming your own boss and getting into something you feel you know enough about, or are interested enough in to learn about. It could be cleaning windows or it could be offering advice or treatment to others. Only you know where your talents lie. Being self employed or working for yourself is extremely interesting, but to start with it may be a bit difficult. Once you have paid all the bills, though, anything left over is yours. If you pay yourself first, you will almost certainly find that there is not enough to pay the bills, but if you're able to strike the right balance then working for yourself will feel great.

If you work hard and get a promotion, bear in mind that the people you had been working with before may not feel you are one of them anymore. This can lead to problems, so make sure you can see your way forward if this happens as otherwise, you might not feel good about it.

Write a Book

Now here's something that a lot more people than you might imagine are doing, thanks to home computers and the internet. Everybody has one book in them, so the saying goes, but most of these books never get out into the light of day as they stay in the mind. This is very often the best place for them, because writing a book that gets published is putting your head above the parapet, and some people like to knock things down! Once you have written a book, it's like a monument to how you thought, or felt as you were writing it. The art of writing is reliant on inspiration and perseverance. The original idea of the book you were going to write may change as you write it.

The reason you should have a go at writing a book, and it does not have to be more than sixty four pages (about twenty thousand words) is not for others, but for yourself. You may write a book and file it away, tell no one about it and feel very good about it.

The act of writing a book is tied up with the journey you will go on as you write it. The ideas that you reject or invent as you go along will be more valuable to you than the finished item. If you actually finish a book and it gets published, you go on another journey and someone, somewhere will be inspired by your work. One of your readers may meet up with someone that otherwise they never would have. More importantly, the best and most exciting things that will come from publishing your book is the meeting that you, the author, will have that would not have happened if you had not started typing!

The subject of your book is something that will come to you. Many people write about things, places and people they know, but this can lead to problems if someone feels they have been portrayed in a poor light. Fiction is a crowded marketplace but is nonetheless a very attractive proposition. Once the muse sits on your shoulder, the words will pour out on some days whereas on others, you will not be able to write a word. So pick a subject or theme and just start, and see what happens.

Yoga

We all read about yoga and its place in the mainstream of modern life. Yoga has steadily brought about a revolution for millions of people, and yet there remains a feeling that it's a bit out of the ordinary. Yoga is so much more than just a way to keep fit in mind and body. The main benefits are to gently improve flexibility and strength, co-ordination, balance, breathing and help to find deep relaxation. You will work on improving the function of the circulatory, digestive and hormonal systems as well as your respiratory system. This will help bring emotional stability and clarity of mind, which will then enable you to more readily deal with stressful situations.

If you are not already practising yoga then talk to your friends, read an article or browse a book and do some research. There are many different types of yoga and you will feel drawn to one type, or a certain class or teacher, without perhaps a really good understanding of why. This is good and should be followed – your intuition will always know best.

Initially, you don't need spend lots of money to get the latest outfits and best mat – just start with something loose and comfy and see what other people use and whether they feel and look right for you, and then move on slowly. Most beginner students will tell you that they got into yoga to relieve back pain or stress, or just to become more flexible.

There are a great series of movements that are perfect for every kind of day, and for every kind of person, so there's every reason to start doing yoga as soon as you can.

Yoga exercises are designed around the idea of moving your body to increase its flexibility so doing a bit, or a lot, of yoga on a regular basis will really help you become much more in tune with your body. You will know when an exercise or series is really working for you and when it isn't and you will learn what it is that makes you feel good.

Zen

It's easy to hang on to the everyday things in your life. It is easy to just keep with your job, relationship or ownership as if your life depends on them. You may be so busy holding onto your own life that you have forgotten to just go with the flow. You are afraid to forge ahead, afraid to let go.

Life is like the flow of a river. Life flows at its own pace, and one source of all of your pain and suffering may be your tendency to go against the flow.

Your job stagnates, relationships break down, ownership dissolves, all because you did not want to let go when it was necessary to let things take their own course. You hung on because change is scary. You hung on because you were worried about the unknown, you hung on because you felt secure if nothing changed. You hung on because you refused to believe that life can never remain the same and you would not accept the transience of everything – you wanted to believe you had power over the material world.

You have to trust life and yourself, because your innermost gut feelings will be right. When you come to a crossroads in your life, or start to wonder if you are doing the right thing, trust your instinct to carry you in the right direction. It is very difficult to allow the world to take you in a particular direction. It requires a tough mental attitude not to do what you would do if you did not have an inner voice advising you to go with the flow.

You do not have enough faith in life. In the business of living, you have lost touch with your inner self. It is easy to lead a life like you are lost in a crowd. You have nobody to place your faith in. You live under the false illusion of having everything under your control. The act of getting things done becomes difficult when you continue to hang on, even after you have tried everything.

This is when you need to learn to let go. Sometimes a relationship is over because you tried too hard to make it work. You didn't let go and let it take its own course. In work or privately, once everything has been done, you must learn to let go and let life take the best course to make you feel good. A certain amount of courage is required but, if you didn't want to try, you would not have read this.

The Best Thing is Freedom

www.ingramcontent.com/pod-product-compliance
Lightning Source LLC
Chambersburg PA
CBHW071719040426
42446CB00011B/2134